Copyright ©
MD

All rights reserved. No part of this publication may be reproduced, distributed, or transmitted in any form or by any means, including photocopying, recording, or other electronic or mechanical methods, without the prior written permission of the publisher, except in the case of brief quotations embodied in critical reviews and certain other noncommercial uses permitted by copyright law.

Table of Contents

Introduction 5
   Contraception and getting pregnant 7
   Lifestyle and fertility 8
   When to get help with fertility 9
   Causes for infertility or reduced fertility 10
   What is unexplained infertility? 11
   All about fertility tests 11
      Tests for men 12
      Tests for women 12
   Fertility treatment 12
Polycystic ovary syndrome (PCOS) 13
   Symptoms 14
   When to see a doctor 15
   Causes 15
   Complications 16
   Diagnosis 17
   Treatment 19
   Lifestyle changes 19
   Medications 20
   Lifestyle and home remedies 22
   What tests do you recommend? 24

What are the long-term health implications of PCOS? 25

What to expect from your doctor 25

What to eat if you have PCOS 26

How does diet affect PCOS? 27

Foods to eat 28

Foods to avoid 31

Other lifestyle changes 32

When to see a doctor 33

Outlook 34

Diet, Exercise, and PCOS 35

Medications 37

    Metformin 37

    Clomid 38

    Letrozole 39

    Gonadotropins 39

    Fertility Procedures 41

    Will You Need an Egg Donor? 42

Recipes for Fertility 43

PCOS-Friendly Cookie Dough Bites 43

Cauliflower Crust Pizza (vegan option) 45

Crab-stuffed avocados 48

Smoked salmon with prawns, horseradish cream & lime vinaigrette 50

Cheesy autumn mushrooms 52

Stuffed courgette rolls 54

Italian-style beef stew 57

Roasted ratatouille chicken 59

Nutty chicken curry 61

Easy chicken casserole 64

Tuna steaks with cucumber relish 67

Basil & lemon chickpeas with mackerel 69

One-pan summer eggs 72

Cranberry pecan baked apples 74

Cranachan 76

Mixed Berry Hormone Balancing Smoothie For Ovulation Support .. 79

Easy Spaghetti Squash with Turkey Meatballs (PCOS) 81

Introduction

Fertility is the quality of being able to produce children. As a measure, the fertility rate is the average number of children that a woman has in her lifetime and is quantified demographically. Fertility is most commonly considered when there is a difficulty or an inability to reproduce naturally, and this is also referred to as infertility. Experiencing infertility is not discriminatory against any particular individual and the phenomenon is widely acknowledged, with fertility specialists available all over the world to provide expertise for assisting mothers and couples who experience difficulties having a baby.

Human fertility depends on factors of nutrition, sexual behaviour, consanguinity, culture, instinct, endocrinology, timing, economics, way of life, and emotions.

Fertility differs from fecundity, which is defined as the potential for reproduction (influenced by gamete production, fertilization and carrying a pregnancy to term) Where a woman or the lack of fertility is infertility while a lack of fecundity would be called sterility.

Fertility is about the ability to get pregnant. More than 8 out of 10 couples where the woman is aged under 40 will get pregnant within one year if they have regular unprotected sex. More than 9 out of 10 couples will get pregnant within 2 years.

Regular, unprotected sex means having sex every 2 to 3 days without using contraception.

You don't need to time having sex only around ovulation. Having vaginal sexual intercourse every 2 to 3 days will give you the best chance of getting pregnant.

Remember it's important for you and your partner to try and keep sex enjoyable by concentrating on each other and your relationship, rather than worrying about conceiving. This will help you limit stress.

Contraception and getting pregnant

Most women use contraception as a safe way to avoid getting pregnant when they are not ready for children. When you stop contraception, it is often because you would like to try for a baby. You can read more about stopping contraception here.

If you have been taking contraception that uses hormones (such as the Pill, the patch, injections) for a long time, you may not know your cycle very well (for example how long it is). This is because the bleed that happens when you move to a new packet of the Pill is not a true period. A true period happens when you ovulate (release an egg from your ovaries) and the Pill prevents ovulation. Read more about how pregnancy works.

If you've stopped taking contraceptives that were based on hormones your periods may be a bit irregular (come at different times of the month) for the first few months while your body gets used to the change in hormone levels.

The Pill does not cause infertility but it may cover up conditions that are linked to infertility because lack of periods is a sign of ovulation problems, endometriosis or PCOS. If you do not have periods anyway, these problems may be missed until you come off contraception.

Lifestyle and fertility

Your fertility is affected by your lifestyle. These are the top lifestyle tips for improving your fertility:

- Don't smoke. Smoking ages your ovaries and your eggs and is linked to lower fertility.
- Cut down on alcohol. Heavy drinking is linked to lower fertility.
- Keep caffeine intake below 200 mg a day.
- Stay active. Being moderately active has been shown to help with fertility
- Stay away from illicit drugs.
- Be a healthy weight.

When to get help with fertility

Infertility is only usually found out when a couple haven't managed to get pregnant. Make an appointment with your GP if you haven't conceived after a year.

You should see your GP sooner if:

- you are over 36 (fertility deceases with age)
- you have a known fertility issue, such as endometriosis (link) or polycystic ovary syndrome (PCOS)
- your partner has a known fertility issue, such as low sperm count
- you are concerned you or your partner may have a medical issue that may be affecting your ability to get pregnant
- you have irregular or no periods.

Your GP will ask you about your lifestyle, general health and medical history. They may ask you questions about:

- any previous pregnancies or children you may have

- how long you have been trying to conceive
- how often you have sex
- how long it has been since you stopped using contraception
- if you take any medication
- your lifestyle and habits.

They may also advise you about the things you can do to improve your chances of getting pregnant and how your partner can improve their fertility.

Causes for infertility or reduced fertility

- Ovulation problems
- Endometriosis
- Poor egg quality
- Polycystic ovarian syndrome (PCOS)
- Fallopian tube problems
- Unexplained infertility
- Poor sperm quality
- Age

- Premature ovarian insufficiency

What is unexplained infertility?

Unexplained fertility is when no reason has been found for a person's fertility problems. In this case you should not be offered any fertility drugs taken by mouth as this does not improve the chances of conceiving naturally. Unexplained fertility is more likely if you are over 36 than if you are under.

If you have been trying to conceive naturally for more than two years (including the year before your fertility tests) you may be offered IVF.

All about fertility tests

If you and your partner have been trying unsuccessfully to get pregnant, you will both be offered fertility tests.

Tests for men

Men should be offered a semen test to measure the quantity and quality of their sperm.

Tests for women

Fertility tests for women may include:

- blood tests to check your hormone levels
- tests (including blood tests) to see how well your ovaries may respond to fertility drugs
- an examination to see whether your fallopian tubes are blocked.

Fertility treatment

This will depend on what's causing the problems and what's available in your local area.

There are three main types of fertility treatment:

- drugs to improve ovulation

- surgery if there are blockages or growths in the reproductive system
- assisted conception – including intrauterine insemination (IUI) and in vitro fertilisation (IVF)

Polycystic ovary syndrome (PCOS)

Polycystic ovary syndrome (PCOS) is a hormonal disorder common among women of reproductive age. Women with PCOS may have infrequent or prolonged menstrual periods or excess male hormone (androgen) levels. The ovaries may develop numerous small collections of fluid (follicles) and fail to regularly release eggs.

The exact cause of PCOS is unknown. Early diagnosis and treatment along with weight loss may reduce the risk of long-term complications such as type 2 diabetes and heart disease.

Symptoms

Signs and symptoms of PCOS often develop around the time of the first menstrual period during puberty. Sometimes PCOS develops later, for example, in response to substantial weight gain.

Signs and symptoms of PCOS vary. A diagnosis of PCOS is made when you experience at least two of these signs:

Irregular periods. Infrequent, irregular or prolonged menstrual cycles are the most common sign of PCOS. For example, you might have fewer than nine periods a year, more than 35 days between periods and abnormally heavy periods.

Excess androgen. Elevated levels of male hormones may result in physical signs, such as excess facial and body hair (hirsutism), and occasionally severe acne and male-pattern baldness.

Polycystic ovaries. Your ovaries might be enlarged and contain follicles that surround the eggs. As a result, the ovaries might fail to function regularly.

PCOS signs and symptoms are typically more severe if you're obese.

When to see a doctor

See your doctor if you have concerns about your menstrual periods, if you're experiencing infertility or if you have signs of excess androgen such as worsening hirsutism, acne and male-pattern baldness.

Causes

The exact cause of PCOS isn't known. Factors that might play a role include:

Excess insulin. Insulin is the hormone produced in the pancreas that allows cells to use sugar, your body's primary energy supply. If your cells become resistant to the action of insulin, then your blood sugar levels can rise and your body might produce more insulin. Excess insulin might increase androgen production, causing difficulty with ovulation.

Low-grade inflammation. This term is used to describe white blood cells' production of substances to fight infection. Research has shown that women with PCOS have a type of low-grade inflammation that stimulates polycystic ovaries to produce androgens, which can lead to heart and blood vessel problems.

Heredity. Research suggests that certain genes might be linked to PCOS.

Excess androgen. The ovaries produce abnormally high levels of androgen, resulting in hirsutism and acne.

Complications

Complications of PCOS can include:

- Infertility
- Gestational diabetes or pregnancy-induced high blood pressure
- Miscarriage or premature birth

- Nonalcoholic steatohepatitis — a severe liver inflammation caused by fat accumulation in the liver
- Metabolic syndrome — a cluster of conditions including high blood pressure, high blood sugar, and abnormal cholesterol or triglyceride levels that significantly increase your risk of cardiovascular disease
- Type 2 diabetes or prediabetes
- Sleep apnea
- Depression, anxiety and eating disorders
- Abnormal uterine bleeding
- Cancer of the uterine lining (endometrial cancer)
- Obesity is associated with PCOS and can worsen complications of the disorder.

Diagnosis

There's no test to definitively diagnose PCOS. Your doctor is likely to start with a discussion of your medical history, including your menstrual periods and weight changes. A physical exam will include checking for signs of excess hair growth, insulin resistance and acne.

Your doctor might then recommend:

A pelvic exam. The doctor visually and manually inspects your reproductive organs for masses, growths or other abnormalities.

Blood tests. Your blood may be analyzed to measure hormone levels. This testing can exclude possible causes of menstrual abnormalities or androgen excess that mimics PCOS. You might have additional blood testing to measure glucose tolerance and fasting cholesterol and triglyceride levels.

An ultrasound. Your doctor checks the appearance of your ovaries and the thickness of the lining of your uterus. A wandlike device (transducer) is placed in your vagina (transvaginal ultrasound). The transducer emits sound waves that are translated into images on a computer screen.

If you have a diagnosis of PCOS, your doctor might recommend additional tests for complications. Those tests can include:

Periodic checks of blood pressure, glucose tolerance, and cholesterol and triglyceride levels

Screening for depression and anxiety

Screening for obstructive sleep apnea

Treatment

PCOS treatment focuses on managing your individual concerns, such as infertility, hirsutism, acne or obesity. Specific treatment might involve lifestyle changes or medication.

Lifestyle changes

Your doctor may recommend weight loss through a low-calorie diet combined with moderate exercise activities. Even a modest reduction in your weight — for example, losing 5 percent of your body weight — might improve your condition. Losing weight may also increase the effectiveness of medications your doctor recommends for PCOS, and can help with infertility.

Medications

To regulate your menstrual cycle, your doctor might recommend:

Combination birth control pills. Pills that contain estrogen and progestin decrease androgen production and regulate estrogen. Regulating your hormones can lower your risk of endometrial cancer and correct abnormal bleeding, excess hair growth and acne. Instead of pills, you might use a skin patch or vaginal ring that contains a combination of estrogen and progestin.

Progestin therapy. Taking progestin for 10 to 14 days every one to two months can regulate your periods and protect against endometrial cancer. Progestin therapy doesn't improve androgen levels and won't prevent pregnancy. The progestin-only minipill or progestin-containing intrauterine device is a better choice if you also wish to avoid pregnancy.

To help you ovulate, your doctor might recommend:

Clomiphene. This oral anti-estrogen medication is taken during the first part of your menstrual cycle.

Letrozole (Femara). This breast cancer treatment can work to stimulate the ovaries.

Metformin. This oral medication for type 2 diabetes improves insulin resistance and lowers insulin levels. If you don't become pregnant using clomiphene, your doctor might recommend adding metformin. If you have prediabetes, metformin can also slow the progression to type 2 diabetes and help with weight loss.

Gonadotropins. These hormone medications are given by injection.

To reduce excessive hair growth, your doctor might recommend:

Birth control pills. These pills decrease androgen production that can cause excessive hair growth.

Spironolactone (Aldactone). This medication blocks the effects of androgen on the skin. Spironolactone can cause birth defects, so effective contraception is required while taking this medication. It isn't recommended if you're pregnant or planning to become pregnant.

Eflornithine (Vaniqa). This cream can slow facial hair growth in women.

Electrolysis. A tiny needle is inserted into each hair follicle. The needle emits a pulse of electric current to damage and eventually destroy the follicle. You might need multiple treatments.

Lifestyle and home remedies

To help decrease the effects of PCOS, try to:

Maintain a healthy weight. Weight loss can reduce insulin and androgen levels and may restore ovulation. Ask your doctor about a weight-control program, and meet regularly with a dietitian for help in reaching weight-loss goals.

Limit carbohydrates. Low-fat, high-carbohydrate diets might increase insulin levels. Ask your doctor about a low-carbohydrate diet if you have PCOS. Choose complex carbohydrates, which raise your blood sugar levels more slowly.

Be active. Exercise helps lower blood sugar levels. If you have PCOS, increasing your daily activity and participating in a regular exercise program may treat or even prevent insulin resistance and help you keep your weight under control and avoid developing diabetes.

Preparing for your appointment

You may be referred to a specialist in female reproductive medicine (gynecologist), a specialist in hormone disorders (endocrinologist) or an infertility specialist (reproductive endocrinologist).

Here's some information to help you get ready for your appointment.

What you can do

List symptoms you've been having, and for how long

List all medications, vitamins and supplements you take, including the doses

List key personal and medical information, including other conditions, recent life changes and stressors

Prepare questions to ask your doctor

Keep a record of your menstrual cycles

For PCOS, some basic questions to ask your doctor include:

What tests do you recommend?

How does PCOS affect my ability to become pregnant?

What medications do you recommend to help improve my symptoms or ability to conceive?

What lifestyle modifications do you recommend to help improve my symptoms or ability to conceive?

What are the long-term health implications of PCOS?

I have other medical conditions. How can I best manage them together?

During your appointment, don't hesitate to ask other questions as they occur to you.

What to expect from your doctor

Your doctor is likely to ask you a number of questions, including:

What are your signs and symptoms? How often do they occur?

How severe are your symptoms?

When did each symptom begin?

When was your last period?

Have you gained weight since you first started having periods? How much weight did you gain, and when did you gain it?

Does anything improve or worsen your symptoms?

Are you trying to become pregnant, or do you wish to become pregnant?

Has your mother or sister ever been diagnosed with PCOS?

What to eat if you have PCOS

Polycystic ovary syndrome is a condition that causes hormonal imbalances and problems with metabolism.

Polycystic ovary syndrome (PCOS) is a common health condition experienced by one out of 10 women of childbearing age. PCOS can also lead to other serious health challenges, such as diabetes, cardiovascular problems, depression, and increased risk of endometrial cancer.

How does diet affect PCOS?

A diet that includes high-fiber foods may benefit people with PCOS.

Two of the primary ways that diet affects PCOS are weight management and insulin production and resistance.

However, insulin plays a significant role in PCOS, so managing insulin levels with a PCOS diet is one of the best steps people can take to manage the condition.

Many people with PCOS have insulin resistance. In fact, more than 50 percent of those with PCOS develop diabetes or pre-diabetes before the age of 40. Diabetes is directly related to how the body processes insulin.

Following a diet that meets a person's nutritional needs, maintains a healthy weight, and promotes good insulin levels can help people with PCOS feel better.

Foods to eat

Research has found that what people eat has a significant effect on PCOS. That said, there is currently no standard diet for PCOS.

However, there is widespread agreement about which foods are beneficial and seem to help people manage their condition, and which foods to avoid.

Three diets that may help people with PCOS manage their symptoms are:

A low glycemic index (GI) diet: The body digests foods with a low GI more slowly, meaning they do not cause insulin levels to rise as much or as quickly as other foods, such as some carbohydrates. Foods in a low GI diet include whole grains, legumes, nuts, seeds, fruits, starchy vegetables, and other unprocessed, low-carbohydrate foods.

An anti-inflammatory diet: Anti-inflammatory foods, such as berries, fatty fish, leafy greens, and extra virgin olive oil, may reduce inflammation-related symptoms, such as fatigue.

The DASH diet: Doctors often recommend the Dietary Approaches to Stop Hypertension (DASH) diet to reduce the risk or impact of heart disease. It may also help manage PCOS symptoms. A DASH diet is rich in fish, poultry, fruits, vegetables whole grain, and low-fat dairy produce. The diet discourages foods that are high in saturated fat and sugar.

A 2015 study found that obese women who followed a specially-designed DASH diet for 8 weeks saw a reduction in insulin resistance and belly fat compared to those that did not follow the same diet.

A healthful PCOS diet can also include the following foods:

- natural, unprocessed foods
- high-fiber foods
- fatty fish, including salmon, tuna, sardines, and mackerel
- kale, spinach, and other dark, leafy greens
- dark red fruits, such as red grapes, blueberries, blackberries, and cherries
- broccoli and cauliflower
- dried beans, lentils, and other legumes
- healthful fats, such as olive oil, as well as avocados and coconuts
- nuts, including pine nuts, walnuts, almonds, and pistachios
- dark chocolate in moderation
- spices, such as turmeric and cinnamon

Researchers looking at a range of healthful diet plans found the following slight differences. For example:

Individuals lost more weight with a diet emphasizing monounsaturated fats rather than saturated fats. An example of this kind of diet is the anti-inflammatory diet, which encourages people to eat plant-based fats, such as olive and other vegetable oils.

People who followed a low-carbohydrate or a low-GI diet saw improved insulin metabolism and lower cholesterol levels. People with PCOS who followed a low-GI diet also reported a better quality of life and more regular periods.

In general, studies have found that losing weight helps women with PCOS, regardless of which specific kind of diet they follow.

Foods to avoid

In general, people on a PCOS diet should avoid foods already widely seen as unhealthful. These include:

Refined carbohydrates, such as mass-produced pastries and white bread.

Fried foods, such as fast food.

Sugary beverages, such as sodas and energy drinks.

Processed meats, such as hot dogs, sausages, and luncheon meats.

Solid fats, including margarine, shortening, and lard.

Excess red meat, such as steaks, hamburgers, and pork.

Other lifestyle changes

Lifestyle changes can also help people with PCOS manage the condition. Research has shown that combining a PCOS diet with physical activity can lead to the following benefits:

weight loss

improved insulin metabolism

more regular periods

reduced levels of male hormones and male-pattern hair growth

lower cholesterol levels

Studies have also found that behavioral strategies can help women achieve the weight management goals that, in turn, help manage PCOS symptoms. These practices include:

- goal-setting
- social support networks
- self-monitoring techniques
- caring for psychological well-being

Reducing stress through self-care practices, such as getting enough sleep, avoiding over-commitment, and making time to relax, can also help a person manage PCOS.

When to see a doctor

Common PCOS symptoms include:

- acne
- extra hair growth
- weight gain, especially around the belly
- oily skin
- irregular periods
- discomfort in the pelvic area
- difficulty getting pregnant

Many people who experience these symptoms may not consider them serious enough to discuss with a doctor. Many people do not seek medical help until they have trouble conceiving.

Anyone experiencing these symptoms should discuss their concerns with a doctor: the sooner they can begin a treatment plan the sooner they can feel better.

Outlook

Although there is currently no cure for PCOS, it is possible for a person to reduce their symptoms and improve their quality of life by adopting a healthful diet and becoming more physically active.

Achieving and maintaining a healthy weight and eating healthful fats, lean proteins, and moderate amounts of low-GI carbohydrates can help a person manage PCOS.

Diet, Exercise, and PCOS

Eating a healthy diet is important for women with PCOS. This is partially due to the higher risk of becoming overweight, and partially due to their bodies' trouble with insulin regulation. Is there any one diet that is best for PCOS? That's a matter of debate.

Some studies have claimed that a low-carb diet is the best one for PCOS, but other studies have not found a low-carb advantage. The most important thing is to make sure your diet is rich in nutrient-rich foods and adequate protein and low on high-sugar foods. Avoiding junk food and processed foods is your best bet.

Fertility-Friendly Eating Tips for PCOS

Eat a bigger breakfast and a smaller dinner.

Include more protein and greens.

When you eat carbohydrates, make them complex carbs (like whole grains and beans).

If you eat sweets or a high carb food, combine it with healthy fats (avocado, olive oil, nuts) or protein to slow down the sugar spike.

Regular exercise has also been found to help with PCOS symptoms. In one study, a combination of regular brisk walking and eating a healthier diet improved menstrual cycle regularity by 50%.

Whether diet and exercise alone will help you conceive isn't clear. However, a healthy lifestyle may help your fertility treatments work better, and it will certainly help you feel better overall. Like weight loss, it's worth the effort if you want to get pregnant.

Medications

Some people with PCOS will need medications to treat the condition and/or to help them conceive.

Metformin

Ask your doctor to test your insulin levels. If you're insulin-resistant, taking the diabetes drug metformin can treat the insulin resistance and may help you lose weight. It may also help you conceive.

Metformin is sometimes prescribed to people with PCOS even if they aren't actually insulin-resistant. Using metformin for PCOS is considered off-label use. However, the drug is relatively safe and may help you conceive. According to the research, metformin may:

- Promote weight loss
- Restart regular menstrual cycles
- Improve the effectiveness of some fertility drugs

- Reduce the rate of miscarriage (in those with repeated miscarriage)

Can metformin alone help you get pregnant? This is unlikely. While earlier research found that metformin increased the odds of a woman ovulating on her own, further studies have not found an increase in pregnancy or live birth rates. In other words, the improvement with ovulation didn't lead to increased fertility.

Clomid

Clomid is the most commonly used fertility drug overall, and also the most commonly used treatment for women with PCOS. Many women with PCOS will conceive with Clomid.

Unfortunately, it's not successful for everyone. Some women with PCOS will experience Clomid resistance. This is when Clomid does not trigger ovulation as expected. Studies have found that a combination of metformin and Clomid may help beat Clomid resistance.

Letrozole

If metformin and Clomid are not successful, your doctor may consider the drug letrozole. Also known by its brand name Femara, it is not a fertility drug but is frequently used as one in women with PCOS. Letrozole is actually a cancer medication. However, studies have found that it may be more effective than Clomid at stimulating ovulation in women with PCOS.

Don't be scared off by the fact that the drug is originally intended as a cancer drug. The side effects are relatively mild, and it has been heavily researched in women trying to conceive.

Gonadotropins

If Clomid or letrozole is not successful, the next step is injectable fertility drugs or gonadotropins. Gonadotropins are made of the hormones FSH, LH, or a combination of the two.

Brand names you may recognize are Gonal-F, Follistim, Ovidrel, Bravelle, and Menopur.

Your doctor may suggest a combination of oral and injectable fertility drugs (for example, Clomid with a trigger shot of LH mid-cycle). Another possibility is a cycle with just gonadotropins.

Or, your doctor may suggest gonadotropins with an IUI (intrauterine insemination) procedure. IUI involves placing specially washed semen directly into the uterus via a catheter. The semen may be from a sperm donor or your partner.

One of the possible risks of gonadotropins is ovarian hyperstimulation syndrome (OHSS). This is when the ovaries overreact to the fertility medication. If untreated or severe, it can be dangerous. Women with PCOS are at a higher risk of developing OHSS.

Your doctor may use lower doses of the injectable fertility drugs to avoid this. Ideally, your doctor should use the lowest effective dose. During treatment, if you have any symptoms of OHSS (such as rapid weight gain, abdominal pain, bloating, or nausea), make sure to tell your doctor.

Fertility Procedures

If gonadotropins are not successful, the next step is IVF (in vitro fertilization) or IVM (in vitro maturation). You've likely already heard of IVF. It involves using injectable fertility drugs to stimulate the ovaries so that they will provide a good number of mature eggs. The eggs are retrieved from the ovaries during a procedure known as an egg retrieval.

Those eggs are then placed together with sperm into Petri dishes. If all goes well, the sperm will fertilize some of the eggs. After the fertilized eggs have had between three and five days to divide and grow, one or two are transferred into the uterus. This procedure is known as an embryo transfer. Two weeks later, your doctor will order a pregnancy test to see if the cycle was a success or not.

As with gonadotropin treatment alone, one of the risks of IVF, especially in women with PCOS, is overstimulation of the ovaries. That's where IVM comes in.

IVM stands for in vitro maturation. Instead of giving you high doses of fertility drugs to force your ovaries to mature many eggs, with IVM you receive either no fertility drugs or very low doses. The doctor retrieves immature eggs from the ovaries, and then mature these eggs in the lab. IVM is not offered at all fertility clinics. This is something to consider when choosing a fertility clinic.

Will You Need an Egg Donor?

It's highly unusual for women with PCOS to require an egg donor, unless there are additional fertility issues at hand, like advanced age. However, women who have had procedures such as ovarian drilling or ovarian wedge resection to treat PCOS may have lower ovarian reserves. In this case, an egg donor may be necessary. This is one reason why surgical treatment for PCOS is not recommended.

Recipes for Fertility

PCOS-Friendly Cookie Dough Bites

So what makes these delicious little bites PCOS-friendly?

Great source of complex carbohydrates (think slower rise and fall in blood sugar for better blood sugar management)

Gluten and dairy-free, vegan

Low in refined sugars (only 3 tbsp of maple syrup for the whole recipe!)

Good source of plant-based protein, healthy fats, fiber and B vitamins

Ingredients

- 1 cup gluten free oat flour I used old fashioned oats and pulsed into a flour using a blender. I used an additional 2 tbsp oat flour.
- 1 can chickpeas, drained and rinsed
- 2 tbsp ground flaxseed
- 2 tbsp coconut oil, melted
- 1 tsp vanilla extract
- 3 tbsp pure maple syrup
- ½ cup dairy-free chocolate chips I used the brand Enjoy Life. Mini chocolate chips would also work great here.
- pinch Himalayan pink sea salt

Instructions

1. Place the oat flour in a medium size mixing bowl. If you need to pulse oats into an oat flour, do this using a food processor or blender and grind into a powder.

2. Next, blend the chickpeas into a paste by adding 4-5 tbsp of water as you blend in a food processor. Once smooth, add to the oat flour.
3. Add in the coconut oil, salt, vanilla extract, flaxseed, and maple syrup. Stir to combine.
4. Fold in the chocolate chips. Using a small stainless steel ice cream scoop, form into individual balls. Store in the refrigerator. These can also be frozen for later use.

Cauliflower Crust Pizza (vegan option)

INGREDIENTS

- 1 small head of cauliflower, cut into florets
- 1/2 cup almond flour
- 1/3 cup shredded cheddar cheese (vegans use plant-based cheese)
- 1 tablespoon grated parmesan cheese (vegans use plant-based cheese)

- 1/2 teaspoon dried oregano
- 1/4 teaspoon dried basil
- 1/4 teaspoon garlic powder
- 1/4 teaspoon black pepper
- 1/4 teaspoon salt, divided
- 2 eggs (vegans use vegan egg alternative)
- Cooking spray
- 1 teaspoon canola oil
- 2 cups kale, chopped
- 1/8 teaspoon crushed red pepper
- 1 cup prepared pizza sauce
- 4 ounces shredded mozzarella cheese (vegans use plant-based cheese)

INSTRUCTIONS

1. Preheat oven to 450 degrees F.
2. Place a medium sized cast iron skillet in oven while it heats.

3. Pulse cauliflower florets in a food processor until it resembles rice. Measure 3 1/2 cups of the riced cauliflower.
4. Place in a microwave safe bowl and cook on high for 6 to 7 minutes. Remove from bowl and wrap in paper towels, pressing to remove excess water. Allow to cool 5 to 10 minutes.
5. In a large bowl, mix cauliflower, almond flour, cheddar and parmesan cheeses, oregano, basil, garlic powder, black pepper, half of salt, and eggs (or alternatives) to form a dough.
6. Remove skillet from oven and spray with cooking spray. Press dough into bottom of skillet. Bake 15 minutes or until crust is golden brown. Remove from oven.
7. While crust cooks, heat oil in a medium sauté pan over medium heat. Add kale and season with remaining salt and crushed red pepper. Sauté 5 minutes or until leaves have softened. Set aside.
8. Top crust with sauce, leaving 1 inch uncovered at edges. Top with mozzarella and kale. Return to oven

and cook 10 more minutes or until cheese is bubbling. Allow to cool slightly before serving.

Crab-stuffed avocados

Prep:10 mins

Easy

Serves 4

Stuffing the cavity of a halved avocado has to be one of the easiest ways to serve it, and this crab filling can be made ahead

Ingredients

- 100g white crabmeat
- 1 tsp Dijon mustard
- 2 tbsp olive oil

- handful basil leaves, shredded with a few of the smaller leaves left whole, to serve
- 1 red chilli , deseeded and chopped
- 2 avocados

Method

STEP 1

To make the crab mix, flake the crabmeat into a small bowl and mix in the mustard and oil, then season to taste. Can be made the day ahead. Add the basil and chilli just before serving.

STEP 2

To serve, halve and stone the avocados. Fill each cavity with a quarter of the crab mix, scatter with a few of the smaller basil leaves and eat with teaspoons.

RECIPE TIPS

TIP

For a cheaper version, mix the same ingredients with some flaked tinned tuna rather than crab.

GOES WELL WITH

Ray with buttery parsley & capers

Smoked salmon with prawns, horseradish cream & lime vinaigrette

Preparation and cooking time

Prep:20 mins

Easy

Serves 2

This stunning starter can be assembled ahead, then topped with dressed leaves just before serving.

Ingredients

- 1 tbsp crème fraîche
- 1 tsp horseradish sauce
- 4 slices smoked salmon
- 10 large cooked prawns, peeled but tails left on

For the salad

- juice 1 lime, finely grated zest of ½
- 1 tsp clear honey
- ½ tsp finely grated fresh root ginger
- 2 tbsp light olive oil
- 2 handfuls small leaf salad

Method

STEP 1

Mix the crème fraîche with the horseradish and a little salt and pepper. For the dressing, whisk the lime juice and zest with the honey, ginger and seasoning, then whisk in the oil. Lay the smoked salmon and prawns on 2 plates, then top with a dollop of the horseradish cream. Toss the salad in most of the dressing and pile on top. Drizzle the remaining dressing around the plate and serve.

GOES WELL WITH

Steak with mushroom puff tartlets

Cheesy autumn mushrooms

Preparation and cooking time

Cook:10 mins

5 mins work

Easy

Serves 4

A low-carb treat, ready in 5 mins

Ingredients

- 4 large field mushrooms
- 100g gorgonzola or other blue cheese, crumbled
- 25g walnuts, toasted and roughly chopped
- 4 thyme sprigs
- knob butter, cut into small pieces
- rocket leaves, to serve

Method

STEP 1

Heat oven to 200C/fan 180C/gas 6. Arrange the mushrooms on a baking tray. Scatter over the cheese, walnuts, thyme sprigs and butter. You can do up to this stage a day in advance.

STEP 2

Pop in the oven and cook for 10 mins until the cheese is melted and the mushrooms are softened. Arrange some rocket leaves on plates and place the mushrooms on top.

GOES WELL WITH

Roast pork with fruity sauce

Stuffed courgette rolls

Preparation and cooking time

Prep:20 mins

Plus marinating

Easy

Makes 24 rolls

Try Gordon Ramsay's take on Italian antipasti - tantalise your palate with this no-cook starter

Ingredients

- 4small courgettes , ends trimmed
- 3-4 tbsp olive oil , plus extra to drizzle
- 3-4 tbsp balsamic vinegar , to drizzle
- 250g tub ricotta
- squeeze lemon juice
- handful fresh basil leaves , chopped
- 50g pine nut , toasted (see Know-how, below)

Method

STEP 1

Slice the courgettes lengthways, using a swivel vegetable peeler – you'll need 24 long strips. Drizzle some of the olive oil and balsamic over two large plates and lay the strips flat, trying not to overlap. Sprinkle with more oil and balsamic, cover and leave to marinate in the fridge for at least 20 mins. Can be prepared up to 6 hrs ahead.

STEP 2

Mix the ricotta with lemon juice and seasoning to taste, then mix in the basil and pine nuts. Place 1 tsp of the ricotta mixture onto one end of a courgette strip and roll up. Repeat until you have used up all the filling. Arrange rolls upright on a plate and grind over some black pepper. Drizzle with a little more oil and balsamic vinegar to serve.

RECIPE TIPS

GORDON'S KNOW-HOW

To toast pine nuts, tip into a hot frying pan – no oil needed – for 2-3 mins, shaking the pan often until the kernels are golden all over. Tip onto a plate and leave to cool.

Italian-style beef stew

Preparation and cooking time

Prep:10 mins

Cook:20 mins

Easy

Serves 4

An easy, superhealthy stew full of vitamin C

Ingredients

- 1 onion, sliced
- 1 garlic clove, sliced
- 2 tbsp olive oil
- 300g pack beef stir-fry strips, or use beef steak, thinly sliced
- 1 yellow pepper, deseeded and thinly sliced
- 400g can chopped tomato

- sprig rosemary, chopped
- handful pitted olives

Method

STEP 1

In a large saucepan, cook onion and garlic in olive oil for 5 mins until softened and turning golden. Tip in the beef strips, pepper, tomatoes and rosemary, then bring to the boil. Simmer for 15 mins until the meat is cooked through, adding some boiling water if needed. Stir through the olives and serve with mash or polenta.

RECIPE TIPS

MAKE IT VEGETARIAN

Leave out the beef and cook 1 chopped aubergine and 1 chopped courgette along with the pepper. Finish by sprinkling over some feta cheese.

Roasted ratatouille chicken

Preparation and cooking time

Prep:25 mins

Cook:25 mins

Ready in 50 minutes

Easy

Serves 4

A classic chicken recipe that will keep the crowds coming back for more

Ingredients

- 1 onion , cut into wedges
- 2 red pepper , seeded and cut into chunks
- 1 courgette , cut into chunks
- 1 small aubergine , cut into chunks
- 4 tomatoes , halved

- 4 tbsp olive oil , plus extra for drizzling
- 4 chicken breasts , skin on
- few rosemary sprigs (optional)

Method

STEP 1

Heat oven to 200C/fan 180C/gas 6. Lay all the vegetables and the tomatoes in a shallow roasting tin. Pour over the olive oil and give everything a good mix round until well coated (hands are easiest for this).

STEP 2

Put the chicken breasts, skin side up, on top of the vegetables and tuck in some rosemary sprigs, if using. Season everything with salt and black pepper and drizzle a little oil over the chicken. Roast for about 35 mins until the vegetables are soft and the chicken is golden. Drizzle with oil before serving.

GOES WELL WITH

Tray-baked potatoes

Nutty chicken curry

Preparation and cooking time

Prep:6 mins

Cook:12 mins

Easy

Serves 4

Fast and flavoursome, this creamy chicken curry is ready in under 20 minutes

Ingredients

- 1 large red chilli , deseeded

- ½ a finger-length piece fresh root ginger, roughly chopped
- 1 fat garlic clove
- small bunch coriander, stalks roughly chopped
- 1 tbsp sunflower oil
- 4 skinless chicken breasts, cut into chunks
- 5 tbsp peanut butter
- 150ml chicken stock
- 200g tub Greek yogurt

Method

STEP 1

Finely slice a quarter of the chilli, then put the rest in a food processor with the ginger, garlic, coriander stalks and one-third of the leaves. Whizz to a rough paste with a splash of water if needed.

STEP 2

Heat the oil in a frying pan, then quickly brown the chicken chunks for 1 min. Stir in the paste for another min, then add the peanut butter, stock and yogurt. When the sauce is gently bubbling, cook for 10 mins until the chicken is just cooked through and sauce thickened. Stir in most of the remaining coriander, then scatter the rest on top with the chilli, if using. Eat with rice or mashed sweet potato.

RECIPE TIPS

USE UP PEANUT BUTTER - PRAWN & NOODLE SALAD

Whisk together 2 tsp peanut butter, 2 tsp sweet chilli sauce and 2 tsp lime juice, then heat through in a frying pan with 150g straight-to-wok rice noodles, a handful cooked prawns, a handful beansprouts and a handful coriander leaves. Serves 1.

USE UP PEANUT BUTTER - SATAY PORK SKEWERS

Thread 500g pork strips onto 8 skewers, then brush with a little oil. Mix 3 tbsp peanut butter with 150ml tub natural yogurt, a squeeze of lime juice and a finely diced red chilli. Grill or griddle the skewers for 2-3 mins, turning, until cooked through. Serve with the satay dipping sauce, rice and a salad. Serves 4.

USE UP PEANUT BUTTER - BANANA BREAKFAST SMOOTHIE

Blend 2 bananas with 400ml milk, 4 tbsp oats, 2 tsp clear honey and 1 tbsp peanut butter. Serves 2.

Easy chicken casserole

Preparation and cooking time

Prep:20 mins

Cook:1 hr

Easy

Serves 4

This flavoursome, low-fat chicken casserole is easy to make and freezes really well, so why not make double and freeze for speedy midweek meals

Ingredients

- 2 tbsp sunflower oil
- 400g boneless, skinless chicken thigh , trimmed and cut into chunks
- 1 onion , finely chopped
- 3 carrots , finely chopped
- 3 celery sticks, finely chopped
- 2 thyme sprigs or ½ tsp dried
- 1 bay leaf , fresh or dried
- 600ml vegetable or chicken stock
- 2 x 400g / 14oz cans haricot beans , drained
- chopped parsley , to serve

Method

STEP 1

Heat the oil in a large pan, add the chicken, then fry until lightly browned. Add the veg, then fry for a few mins more. Stir in the herbs and stock. Bring to the boil. Stir well, reduce the heat, then cover and cook for 40 mins, until the chicken is tender.

STEP 2

Stir the beans into the pan, then simmer for 5 mins. Stir in the parsley and serve with crusty bread.

GOES WELL WITH

Classic white loaf

Tuna steaks with cucumber relish

Preparation and cooking time

Prep:15 mins

Cook:3 mins - 4 mins

Easy

Serves 4

Good source of heart-healthy omega-3 fatty acids

Ingredients

- 3 tbsp olive oil
- 4 tuna steaks, about 140g/5oz each
- For the relish
- ½ cucumber
- 2 spring onions, finely chopped
- 1 medium tomato, finely chopped
- ½ large red chilli, seeded and finely chopped

- 1tbsp olive oil
- 2tbsp chopped parsley
- 1tbsp lime or lemon juice

Method

STEP 1

Put the oil into a food bag and add the tuna steaks. Rub well together and leave for 30 mins while you make the relish. Peel the cucumber, halve lengthways and scoop out the seeds. Chop the flesh into a small dice. Mix with the rest of the ingredients, seasoning to taste. Set aside.

STEP 2

To griddle: heat the pan to hot, then cook the steaks, turning after 2 mins, and cooking for another 2 mins each side depending on the thickness of the steaks. Meaty fish is best served slightly 'pink'. Remove the steaks from the heat allow to stand for 3-5 mins, then spoon over the relish and serve.

RECIPE TIPS

TO BBQ

When the grill is ready to cook, remove the fish from the bag, dabbing off excess oil. Season and cook for barely 2 mins each side.

GOES WELL WITH

Classic potato salad

Basil & lemon chickpeas with mackerel

Preparation and cooking time

Prep:10 mins

Cook:15 mins

Easy

Serves 4

Good Food favourite Lesley Waters proves that healthy can be hearty - and tasty too!

Ingredients

- 3 tbsp olive oil , plus extra for drizzling
- 1 bunch spring onion , sliced
- 1 large garlic clove , crushed
- zest 1 lemon and squeeze of juice
- 2 x 400g can chickpeas , drained and rinsed
- 150ml vegetable stock
- 85g SunBlush tomato , halved
- 4 mackerel fillets, skin on
- 1 large bunch basil

Method

STEP 1

Heat 2 tbsp oil in a large, shallow pan. Add the spring onions, garlic and lemon zest, then cook for 2 mins until the onions are tender but still very green. Add the chickpeas, then stir until well coated in the onion mixture. Lightly crush with a potato masher, then add the stock and tomatoes. Simmer for 3-4 mins or until the liquid is absorbed, then set aside to cool slightly.

STEP 2

Meanwhile, heat the remaining oil in a large, non-stick frying pan over a medium heat. Season the mackerel fillets on both sides and fry for 3 mins each side, starting on the skin side. You'll probably need to cook these in two batches.

STEP 3

Add the basil and a squeeze of lemon juice to the chickpeas, then season to taste. To serve, spoon the warm chickpeas onto serving plates, drizzle with a little extra olive oil and top with the mackerel fillets.

GOES WELL WITH

Apricot & raspberry buckle

One-pan summer eggs

Preparation and cooking time

Prep:5 mins

Cook:12 mins

Easy

Serves 2

Satisfy your hunger with this fresh and easy vegetarian supper, or brunch if you prefer

Ingredients

- 1 tbsp olive oil

- 400g courgettes (about 2 large ones), chopped into small chunks
- 200g/7oz pack cherry tomatoes , halved
- 1 garlic clove , crushed
- 2 eggs
- few basil leaves , to serve

Method

STEP 1

Heat the oil in a non-stick frying pan, then add the courgettes. Fry for 5 mins, stirring every so often until they start to soften, add the tomatoes and garlic, then cook for a few mins more. Stir in a little seasoning, then make two gaps in the mix and crack in the eggs. Cover the pan with a lid or a sheet of foil, then cook for 2-3 mins until the eggs are done to your liking. Scatter over a few basil leaves and serve with crusty bread.

RECIPE TIPS

TIP

No fresh basil? Simply stir a couple of teaspoons of pesto into the pan before adding the eggs.

MAKE IT FOR BRUNCH

All-in-one full English Counts as 2 of 5-a-day Fry 2 rashers back bacon in the oil until crisp, then replace the courgettes with a handful sliced mushrooms. Add the tomatoes (omit the garlic) and eggs, then finish off the recipe as before.

GOES WELL WITH

Chillied cheese on toast

Cranberry pecan baked apples

Preparation and cooking time

Total time 20 mins

Ready in about 20 minutes

Easy

Stuffed baked apples that taste as good as they look - and they're super healthy

Ingredients

- cooking apples
- dried cranberries
- pecans , chopped or whole
- oranges , finely grated zest and juice

Method

STEP 1

Heat oven to 200C/180C fan/gas 6. Core cooking apples, fill their centres with dried cranberries, chopped or whole pecans and the finely grated zest and juice of oranges, then bake until tender (which should take about 20 mins).

Cranachan

Preparation and cooking time

Prep:15 mins

Cook:5 mins

Easy

Serves 4

Sweet summer raspberries folded into cream flavoured with honey, whisky and toasted oatmeal - what could be more delicious?

THE BEST RANCH EVER

INGREDIENTS

- 1 egg
- 1 cup of avocado oil or light olive oil
- ½ tsp mustard powder
- ½ tsp onion powder
- 1 tsp garlic powder
- 1 tbsp chives
- 1 tbsp dill
- 2 tbsp red wine vinegar

INSTRUCTIONS

If using a stick blender:

1. Add all ingredients into a mason jar
2. Use a stick blender to emulsify

If using a food processor:

1. Add only 2 tablespoons of oil to food processor. Reserve the rest for later.
2. Add the rest of the ingredients into the food processor.
3. Turn the food processor 'on' Once all of the ingredients have mixed, begin slowly drizzling oil into the food processor.

If using a whisk:

1. Add only 2 tablespoons of oil to your bowl. Reserve the rest for later.
2. Add the rest of the ingredients into the bowl.
3. Whisk all of the ingredients together well, and then while actively and violently whisking begin very, very slowly drizzling oil into the bowl. This should take you a couple of minutes.

Mixed Berry Hormone Balancing Smoothie For Ovulation Support

Support ovulation -- arguably the most important part of the female cycle -- with this mixed berry hormone balancing smoothie! It utilizes the wisdom of seed cycling to promote healthy detoxification of estrogen, helping to regulate headaches, mood swings, and more.

Course Beverage

Cuisine American

Prep Time 5 minutes

Servings 1

Calories 341 kcal

Ingredients

- 2 leaves kale exclude stems

- 1 cup frozen berries blueberries, strawberries, blackberries, and/or raspberries
- 1 tablespoon sunflower seeds preferably soaked and dehydrated first
- 1 tablespoon flax seed meal
- 1/2 banana or 1/2 avocado
- 1 teaspoon maca powder
- 2 cups almond milk
- 1/2 teaspoon vanilla extract

Instructions

1. Combine all ingredients and blend well for 20 to 30 seconds.
2. Serve right away.

Easy Spaghetti Squash with Turkey Meatballs (PCOS)

Prep Time:

15 minutes

Cook Time:

1 hour

Servings:

5

INGREDIENTS

- 1 pound organic ground turkey
- 1 onion (finely chopped)
- 3 cloves garlic (minced)
- 1 shallot (diced)
- 1 cup oats (coarsely ground)
- 1/2 teaspoon garlic powder
- 1/2 teaspoon oregano

- 1 teaspoon sea salt
- 1/2 teaspoon black pepper
- 2 eggs (lightly beaten)
- 1/4 cup water
- 1/4 cup fresh parsley (chopped)
- 1 large spaghetti squash
- 1 cup water
- 1 tablespoon olive oil
- sea salt and black pepper, to taste
- 1 jar Boutique-brand marinara sauce – I like Rao's. You want to find a sauce that uses olive oil, is low in sugar and natural ingredients
- 1 8 ounce can organic tomato sauce (I like Muir Glen)
- 1 14.5 ounce can organic diced tomatoes (I like Muir Glen)
- 1 tablespoon olive oil
- 1/2 cup onion (chopped)
- 1/2 cup green bell pepper (chopped)
- 2 cloves garlic (minced)
- 8 ounce baby spinach or baby kale

- fresh parsley and/or basil, to garnish

INSTRUCTIONS

1. Combine all ingredients (above the spaghetti squash) and mix by hand to combine. Roll 1 1/2" meatballs and place on a baking drying rack that has been placed on a foil covered baking sheet. Bake at 375 for about 25-30 minutes.

2. Cut squash in half lengthwise and scoop out seeds. Place cut side down in a baking dish. Prick top with fork or knife. Add water to pan and bake at 375 for 30 minutes. The squash is done when you can easily slide a fork through. Don't over cook or the squash will be mushy. Scrape the squash strands into a bowl and add olive oil and salt and pepper to taste.

3. Heat olive oil in a heavy large pan or Dutch oven. Add onion, pepper and garlic and cook until fragrant and tender.

4. Add marinara, tomato sauce and diced tomatoes and bring to a simmer.

5. Add cooked meatballs and simmer for about 20 minutes.

6. Add spinach and cook until just wilted.

7. Serve over spaghetti squash and garnish with parsley and basil.

NUTRITION INFORMATION

Per Serving: Calories: 424; Total Fat: 24 g; Saturated Fat: 5 g; Monounsaturated Fat: 5 g; Polyunsaturated Fat: 1 g; Cholesterol: 153mg; Sodium: 1790 mg; Potassium: 832 mg; Carbohydrate: 27 g; Fiber: 6 g; Sugar: 12 g; Protein: 26 g

Nutrition Bonus: Vit A: 121%; Vit C : 96%; Iron:30%; Calcium: 15%;